I0412782

The
Up's and Downs
of
TINA'S LIFE

JOANN MOSCHGAT

Order this book online at www.trafford.com
or email orders@trafford.com

Most Trafford titles are also available at major online book retailers.

Printed in the United States of America.

ISBN: 978-1-4669-4291-2 (sc)
ISBN: 978-1-4669-4290-5 (e)

Library of Congress Control Number: 2012910415

Trafford rev. 08/09/2012

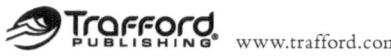 www.trafford.com

North America & International
toll-free: 1 888 232 4444 (USA & Canada)
phone: 250 383 6864 ✦ fax: 812 355 4082

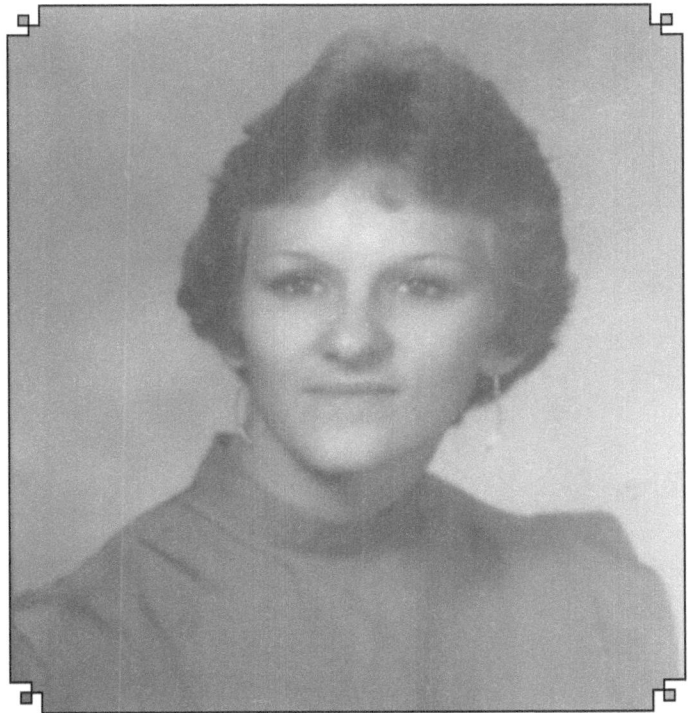

Tina Marie Moschgat's life began on August 2, 1967. Tina was a beautiful bundle of joy weighing 5 pounds 6 ounces and had the curliest hair you have ever seen. Tina

was born in Johnstown Pa. to Joan and George Moschgat, the town was a rural city totaling 6.1 miles. Johnstown was a place to raise a family, a place where everyone knew everyone and nothing ever happened, until Tina came into the world.

Tina was the baby of the family; she had two brothers Andrew 3 and George age 11 months. Tina was a very good baby, then she turned two and it was a challenging life for her after that. Tina's life was filled with events that made anyone wonder how she survived and was still the most joyful person you would have ever wanted to know. She could light up a room with her very presence. Tina was a tomboy from the start; she loved to follow her brothers.

Outside is where Tina loved to be, she was the kind of child that if you took your eyes off her for two seconds she would get into mischief. Tina was four and this began her courageous life. On a day like any other Tina was outside playing with Andrew and other friends, when all of a sudden she ran across the road and was hit by a car doing fifty miles an hour and flew fifty feet into a stack of wood that sat in front of the house. The speed limit was only twenty five miles an hour and not even heavily

traveled. Tina had suffered severe brush burns over ninety five percent of her body.

Tina was in the hospital for a week following the accident where she could not wear any clothes due to the severity of the burns. She had to undergo daily painful cleaning of the burns for several months. Tina took it all in stride, and recovered with no outward scars but she now knew to look both ways before crossing the road.

Tina was the kind of person who always had a lot of friends, at the age of five Tina and two of her friends went up the railroad tracks to a tree vine where they enjoyed swinging on it.

One of the girls climbed on the vine with Tina. Tricia was one of the friends that was with her and she's the one that climbed on the vine with her. When she climbed on the vine with Tina the vine broke and they fell to the ground. Tricia landed on top of Tina knocking her unconscious, Tricia and Robbie the other friend carried Tina about a quarter mile to get her help not realizing the severity of Tina's injury. These two brave children took her to Tricia's house because they knew Tina's mother was at work, Tina's mothers office was right up the street from their home.

Tricia's mother took Tina to her mother at work; the paramedics were waiting when they arrived. The paramedic's noticed there was a bone sticking out of Tina's arm, they took Tina to the hospital where her arm had to be reset and they put her in a full arm cast.

Now when Tina was six she was outside playing with her brother George who picked up an axe and began swinging it around, unfortunately Tina was behind him and George not realizing this hit her in the forehead splitting her eye open. Once again Tina was being rushed to the hospital to have stitches. The doctor said Tina was very lucky that she didn't lose her eye.

Later that summer Tina was at the park with her family swimming she got stung by a bee, again she was rushed to the hospital because she was going into anaphalatic shock.

Tina was active and was loved by all who knew her. One day when Tina was seven she had a discussion with her mother that did not go her way, so Tina packed her bags and climbed out her window and went next-door to her longtime childhood friend Tracy. Tina's mother knew right where Tina was and knew that she would decide to come home when she was ready.

Every summer growing up Tina went to Uncle Steve and Aunt Barbara's house, they had a daughter Stephanie and Tina considered her thru life to be one of her best friends. Tina would go on trips with them also. One summer day Tina and Stephanie was walking around town, and Tina found a dead rat on the sidewalk and picked it up and threw it into someone's car, of course they got a laugh out of it, but when her uncle and aunt found out what happened, she also got a spanking.

So at the age of eight her mother decided to send her to Catholic school until she improved some but Tina never stopped being Tina, she continued with her devilish childish acts.

Tina had energy about her, she thrived for new adventures. For example Tina and Tracy at the age of ten walked to the next town known as Devils Hollow. This was a neighborhood where it was known to be a party spot.

Tina and Tracy started going to a man's house who lived in Devils Hollow every day. One day Tina's mother came home from work early to find her daughter not home, so she asked the neighbors if they had seen her. Joan then found out that she was hanging out with a man twice her

age. Joan then went to the man's house to see if she was there, but Tina being Tina snuck out the back door. They called the man Shark and Tina was head over heels for him and enjoyed hanging out with him. Joan of course knowing the man was twenty years old was not going to have her daughter part of that.

Tina however was not going to take her mother's advice to go near him again, she still continued to see him for a long time. Joan had finally reached her breaking point Joan told Shark that if she ever seen her daughter near him again she would call the authorities and have him put in jail, Shark moved away shortly after that.

Joan said good riddens, things seemed to get better for Tina. Her mother received a promotion at work and was able to do more things with the kids.

Joan took the children to Daytona Beach as usual every summer. August 2, was Tina's birthday so they had a party on the beach, on the way back home they stopped at South of the Border, South Carolina to celebrate George's birthday since his is August 7th. Tina, George, Andrew, and Tracy went to the pool that hot August morning before heading back home.

Tina was a remarkable swimmer and diver so of course as soon as the kids got to the pool Tina headed for the board. Tina was in preparation for one of her perfect dives as she jumped up and down on the board, something went wrong she slipped from the board and hit her head and neck on the diving board. She went to the bottom of the pool no one knew what had happened as everyone was watching to see if she was ok.

The children panicked as they were yelling for help. A woman who happened to be a 75 year old nurse from New Jersey heard them and dove in and rescued her from the pool, Tina was unconscious the nurse told the kids to call 911 and notify Joan of what just had happened.

Tina was rushed to the hospital with her mom in the ambulance. Joan was waiting for the hospital staff to tell her what she feared hearing that her child was paralized from the chest down. Joan was then notified by the doctor that they were putting a halo on her head and that she had broken her neck. Joan watched as her prescious child had holes drilled in the sides of her skull so the halo could be then placed on her head.

Tina's and Joan's life would never be the same. The two of them would forever need each other; Tina and her mom

were in the hospital in South Carolina for two long weeks. Tina was then flown by helicopter with a doctor, nurse and her mom to a hospital in Pittsburgh, Pa close to her home where she would go thru several months of rehab, now having to learn to live life as a quadriplegic. Tina would be in a wheelchair for the rest of her life, but never once did she even allow this accident to bring her down.

Tina amazed everyone with her spirits and drives to get home, and she made it. There would have to be changes done to her home to allow her the space she would need to move around in a chair, Tina would also have nurses to care for her needs. Joan would learn how to take care of her daughter until they could find a nurse, which they did find a wonderful woman who cared for her personal needs, her name was Doris and she cared for Tina for 13 years.

Andrew her older brother would also be her left arm for a long time taking her where she needed to go. Tina went back to school and graduated with her class, she continued her journey in life no differently except for her sitting and not standing, she was still herself. That wild girl, the one who everyone was drawn to, never allowing her being in a wheelchair to get in her way.

Tina started dating like all young girls do, she met a guy named Bill who became her first boyfriend. Tina and Bill were together for a short time when a tragic accident happened and he lost his life in a fire. Tina was strong and got thru her loss; she continued her life and dated again eventually. Tina had like all young girls loves come and go until she met her true love who she would spend the rest of her life with, his name was Tom but everyone called him Tucker.

Tina and Tucker had ups and downs in their relationship as all do but they were happy, he ended up moving in with Tina and her family at age sixteen, he had some family issues at home. Tina was thrilled to have him there, her mom not so much but she got over it seeing how happy she was. Tina and Tucker had plans for forever future, and they succeeded in a life that would fulfill all their dreams. Tina and Tucker wanted to start a family, they had finally reached a time in their life when they did just that.

Tina and Tucker had taken a trip to Niagara Falls for their anniversary in 1997, it was then they conceived their son who was born October 1, 1998. Mitchel Thomas was to be his name and was the center of their lives, Tina loved being a mother it made her family complete.

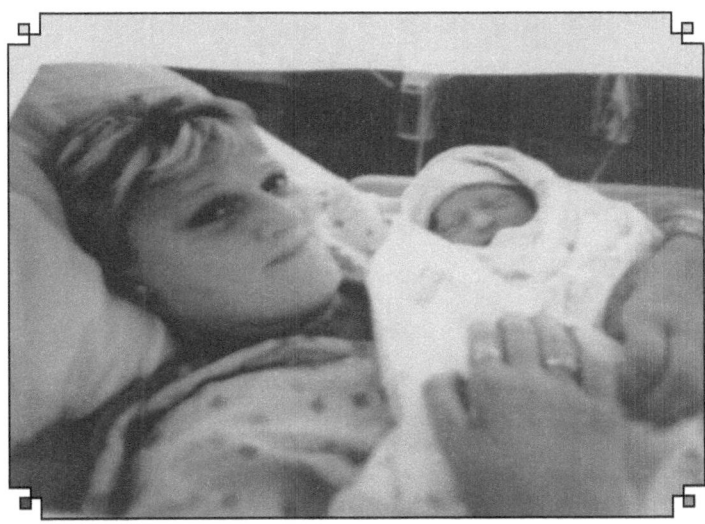

TINA'S FAVORITE PICURE IN THE WHOLE WORLD

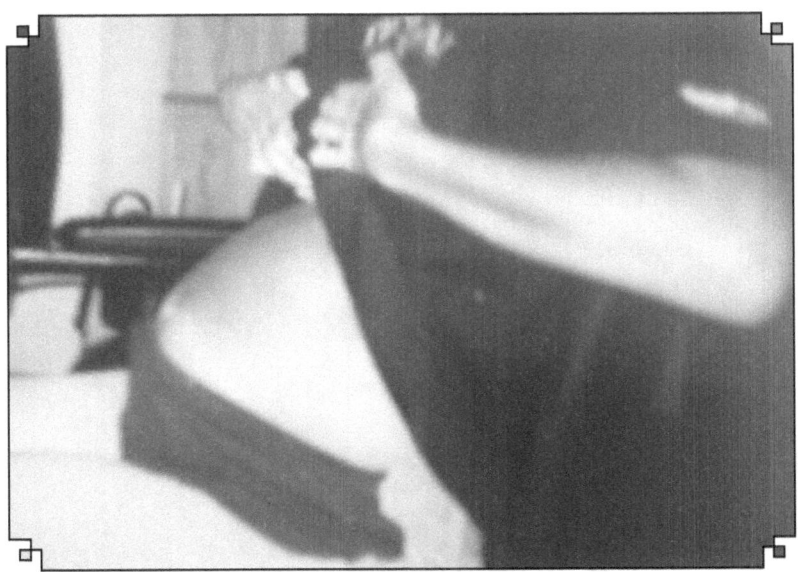

BABY MITCHEL IN HERE

Tina and Tucker decided after Mitchel was born that they wanted to raise their family in Tampa, Florida. Tina was

now thirty one, life could not have been better. Tina and her family would go to the beach every weekend, she loved the sun, sand and surf everything Florida had to offer. There were times when Tina and Tucker had time to themselves, where they would spend time with friends at their favorite hangout shooting pool. She was known to be a pool shark. Mitchel of course was not left out he was able to spend quality time with nunnie. Joan enjoyed this time with him because Tina wanted Mitchel to know everything about her and her family and Joan like all grandmothers cherished time with him.

Time went on as time does, Tina and the family found a place they loved in Brandon, Florida. This was where Home would be for the rest of her life. She was only thirty two at this time, she was very happy because now she could be the mother and homemaker she had wanted to be. She was able to cook for her family as this was a passion of hers. Friends and family would come over just for her food.

She could now have parties for every holiday, birthdays, or just too hang out with friends. Tina took control as she always did because nothing would get in the way of her independence to do want she wanted when she wanted to.

Tina also had other loves, she loved to oil paint and this is quite an accomplishment for anyone to be able to do but she did it with passion, from the heart.

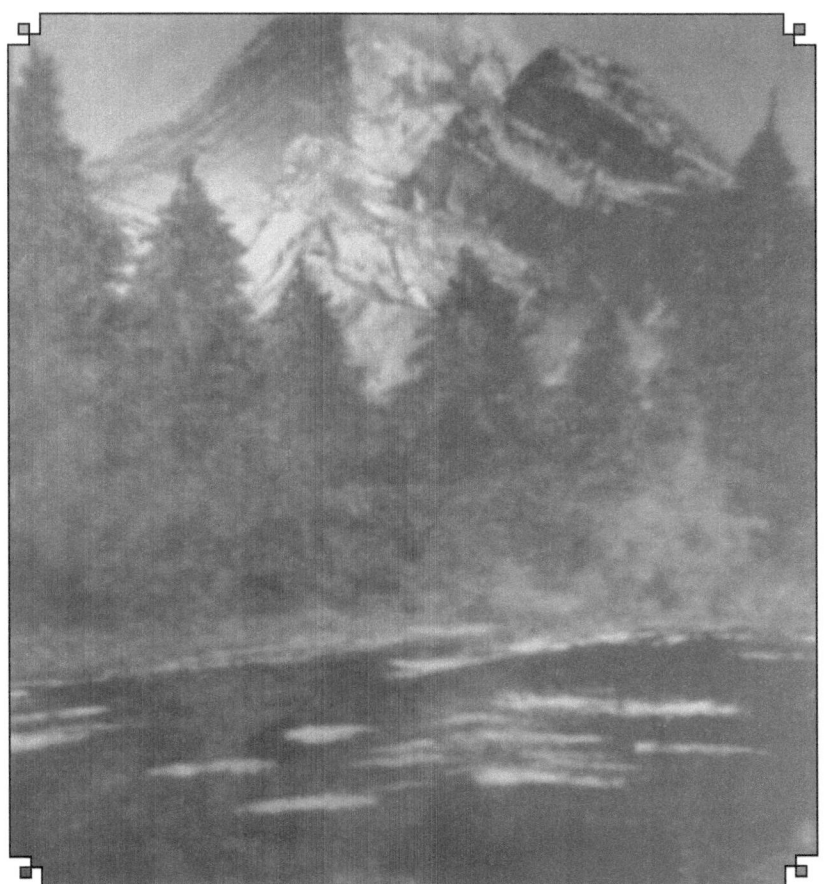

TINA'S FIRST PAINTING

Tina also loved her boat because being on the water was where she felt free.

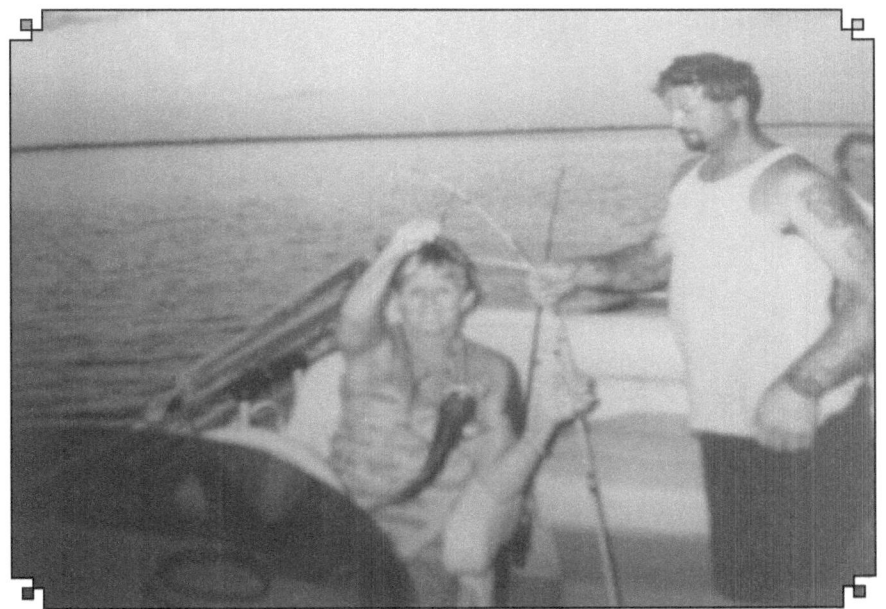

THE GANG SHARK FISHING

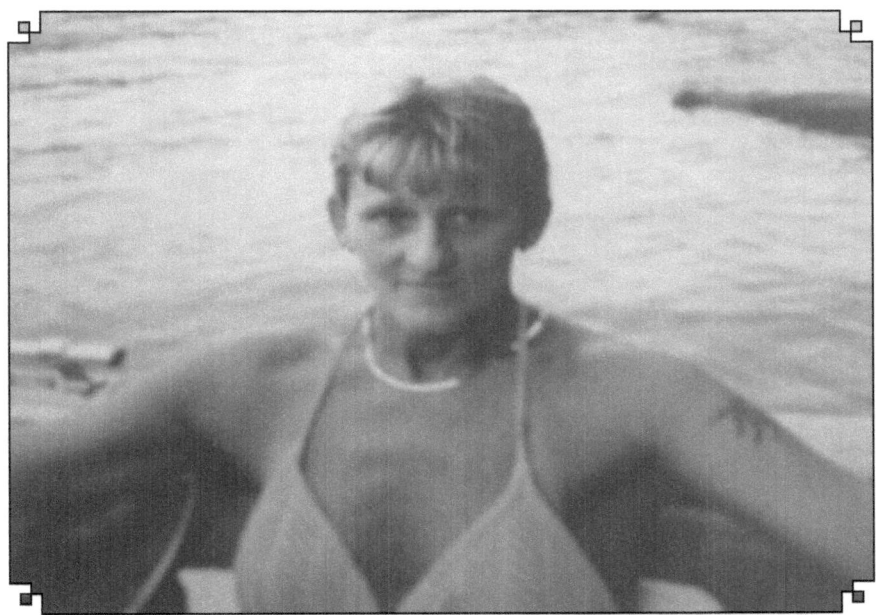

TINA SUNBATHING

Tina would take Mitchel fishing from a young age,

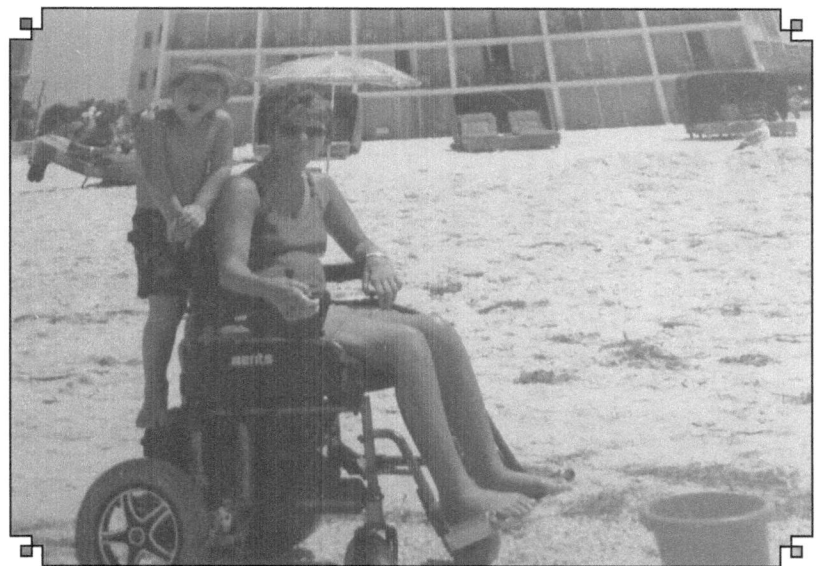

FAMILY VACATION AT BEACH

She would go camping with him and his friends as she was known as the mother of the neighborhood. As Mitchel grew up birthdays were very important around Tina's home, she at one time had a petting zoo, magicians, clowns, water slides. Tina would always go over and beyond to make Mitchel as happy as she was, she would give Mitchel the best of everything life had too offer.

Tina loved to travel; she wanted to show Mitchel the world and his own back yard. They went too amusement parks, water parks, the zoo, the aquarium, because these were times that Tina enjoyed and always captured everything on film.

Tina was always taking pictures even when you would least expect. Pictures filled her home; anyone that walked into her home could see her passion for family, friends and great adventures. Tina's vacations were like no other just to name a few, she went to the Bahamas, St. Kitts, Mexico, and Las Vegas, she went to the Hoover Dam and took helicopter ride over the Grand Canyon. But this was not her first helicopter ride; Tina had also flown over the volcanos of Hawaii and also flew over Niagara Falls. There was one vacation that Tina and Tucker were on in Aruba, they decided to rent a four-wheel drive vehicle for the day.

Things turned bad however, the vehicle they were driving broke down, Tina told Tucker to go for help but he said he would not leave her. So what Tucker did was amazing, he picked her up and carried her for a few miles in the hot desert sands. Tina's vacations like her life were always filled with drama and adventure.

Tina had many friends but she had one true friend that she could entrust anything, her name was Danielle.

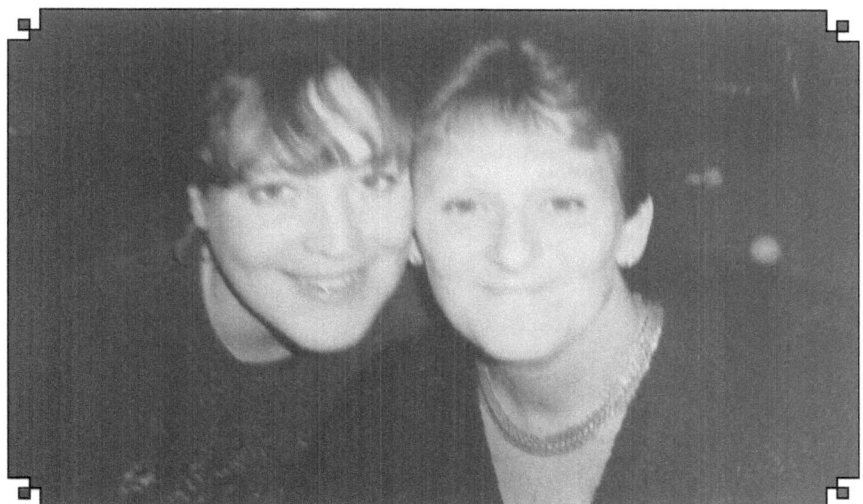

DANIELLE AND TINA

Danielle became like one of the family, their kids played and grew up together, Danielle's son Shane became Mitchel's long time friend. Tina would take Shane everywhere with them, they were like brothers and Tina treated him as if he was her own.

Tina had two other close friends Carrie and Jill. Jill and Tina's relationship was personal and professional it was one they would hold onto.

Tina hired Jill in 2004. Jill became a close friend of the family, now that's not to say that they always saw eye to eye on everything but who does. Tina would invite her to parties and other family functions that she had. During Jill's time

there Jill became pregnant and when the baby was born Tina welcomed him as well. Tina went to the baby shower and even to the hospital when the baby was born. Tina's love of all children filled her home at any given time.

One time one of Mitchel's friends needed help in a big way, Tina opened her home her heart and her loving arms for this child as she would do for any child in need. Tina bought him whatever he needed and never asked for anything in return.

Tina would do this for anyone who was in need because her love for people would move her to go out of her way. She would give you the shirt off her back if she thought you needed it more than her. Her love didn't stop there she loved animals as well, she always had pets in her home whether it be birds, cats, dogs or fish.

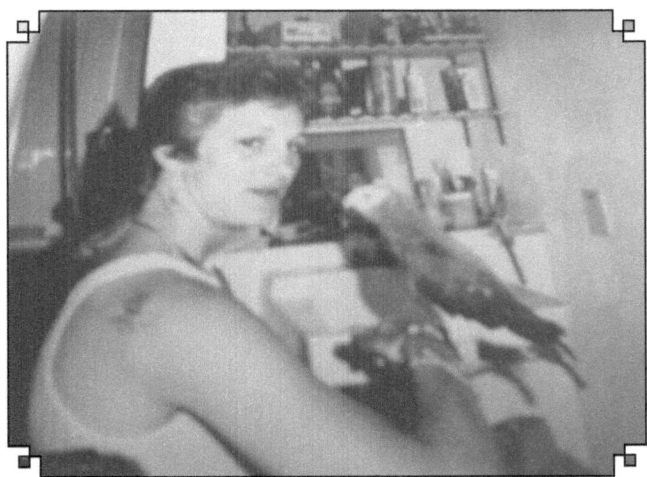

She also loved to shop, people at the stores she went to even knew her by name. Tina was always on the go, she did not like to stay at home when she could be out enjoying the world with the ones she loved.

It was the summer of 2009 when Tina started to get sick, it was then that she was told she had bladder cancer. Life for Tina became a bit more challenging; she now had to undergo treatments for the cancer on weekly basis. By 2010 Tina was told the cancer was in remission, she was relieved that her bladder did not have to be removed.

Tina was also told that the type of cancer she had was a fast growing carcinoma and the chance of it coming back was very high. She had to go for checkups every six months, but she did not let this get her down in anyway. Tina still lived her life to the fullest every day. In December 2010 she had a follow up and she found out the cancer was back.

Andrew her older brother was made aware of her condition and made a decision to transfer his government job from California to Florida to spend the last three months of her life with him. Starting April 2011 Tina was in and out of the hospital for several different issues that stemmed from the cancer. Tina also had stage four kidney disease, and

in May of that year due to an experimental chemotherapy treatment she went into renal failure and was in the ICU for ten days with tubes in her back to help the kidneys, this was just the beginning of the last months of her life.

Trips to the hospital became frequent due to all the things cancer did to her body. Tina knew one thing for sure a hospital is not where she wanted to be, so she made a decision to sign up for hospice which is a program that would allow her to stay home with her family and out of the hospitals.

Tina never let it get her down, she loved life, Tina lived everyday those last months knowing that she was dying. Tina wanted more than ever to never miss a moment, she looked at her life and wanted to never forget one moment. She enjoyed her family and wanting to spend as much of that with her son.

Tina went camping with him every weekend because that was one of their favorite things to do, but she invited everyone of his friends and hers, you could say it was her way of celebrating their life together. She enjoyed watching him ride his dirt bike and playing in the mud, she also enjoyed watching her friends enjoy themselves as she captured every moment for what it was and filmed every step.

Tina had that spirit and energy that filled everything she loved and touched. On night of November 30th she told Tucker that she knew something was wrong, and that all she wanted was to make it through Mitchel's birthday. Tina did make it thru Mitchel's birthday, but that was her last conscious day.

Tina was never alone she was surrounded by her family and friends. Tina's mom and friend Jill cared for her as they always did every day all the way till her last day. Brothers Andrew and George never left her side they were with us till the end as well as Danielle and her children.

Aunt Barbara and Uncle Steve came from Pennsylvania unexpectantly for a visit, Thank God for all they did, they were with us from morning till night consoling Tina and me and Mitchel. I am so grateful for family, couldn't have made it without their help. Tina lost her battle to Cancer October 3, 2011.

This was not the end though; as Tina's life came in with a bang she also went out with one to. Tina had two viewings scheduled because she had so many friends not all could fit in one. Flowers from all over filled the funeral home; she

was wearing her favorite color purple in the casket that was chosen by her family.

Tina was taken from the funeral home in a beautiful white hurst to her church where a beautiful mass took place, there was not one dry eye in church. Andrew her older brother and Jill spoke the words from the old and new testament. From there she had a procession where everybody followed her back to the cemetery where the priest blessed her casket, and her son before she was put to rest in her crypt.